THE INTEGRATION OF THE
ENDOCRINE SYSTEM

THE INTEGRATION OF THE ENDOCRINE SYSTEM

BEING THE FIFTH
HORSLEY MEMORIAL LECTURE
DELIVERED AT UNIVERSITY COLLEGE
HOSPITAL MEDICAL SCHOOL
BY

SIR WALTER LANGDON-BROWN
M.D., F.R.C.P.

*Emeritus Professor of Physic in the University of
Cambridge and Consulting Physician
to St Bartholomew's Hospital*

CAMBRIDGE
AT THE UNIVERSITY PRESS
1935

CAMBRIDGE
UNIVERSITY PRESS

University Printing House, Cambridge CB2 8BS, United Kingdom

Published in the United States of America by Cambridge University Press, New York

Cambridge University Press is part of the University of Cambridge.

It furthers the University's mission by disseminating knowledge in the pursuit of education, learning and research at the highest international levels of excellence.

www.cambridge.org
Information on this title: www.cambridge.org/9781107673588

© Cambridge University Press 1935

First published 1935
Re-issued 2014

A catalogue record for this publication is available from the British Library

ISBN 978-1-107-67358-8 Paperback

THE INTEGRATION OF THE ENDOCRINE SYSTEM

I still well remember, almost as if it were yesterday, the thrill of excitement which went through the Physiological Laboratory at Cambridge when on January 30th, 1892, a paper appeared entitled "Remarks on the Function of the Thyroid Gland; a critical and historical review". It was by Victor Horsley, whose name up till then was only known to me by a drawing he made for Schäfer's *Histology*. We eagerly awaited the second part of that paper which appeared a week later. Instinctively we felt that the door was open to a long avenue of discovery. And we were right.

Papers like that do not come out of the blue. Horsley had been working at the subject since 1884. It is perhaps worth while briefly to recall the steps which led up to that paper.

We all know that the story begins with Gull's description of the "cretinoid state" in 1873, which four years later Ord christened myxoedema. In 1882 Kocher and Reverdin independently noted a similar condition following thyroidectomy for goitre, but attributed it to damage to the trachea. Next year, however, hearing of the English cases of myxoedema, they concluded that the removal of the gland was responsible, but only by damage to nerves. In that year the Clinical Society of London appointed a committee to investigate the subject, and of this committee Horsley was a member. His share was to investigate by experiment, for which his training as a physiologist and a surgeon equipped him admirably. It is of interest to note that his first impression led him to say "the question arises whether we have not to do with the simple case of total removal of an excretory organ". Looking at the bloated appearance of a patient with myxoedema, one can easily understand that impression. A similar idea was enunciated in 1892 by Abelous and Langlois as to the function of the adrenals on slighter grounds. But Rolleston on reviewing the evidence in his Goulstonian Lectures in 1895 suggested that Addison's disease was an atony due to the loss of an internal secretion, a few months before Schäfer and Oliver prepared an active adrenal extract. From all this we can see how slow was Claude

Bernard's conception of internal secretion to permeate physiology and medicine. Even when Schiff in 1884 showed the benefits conferred by transplantation of a thyroid into a thyroidectomised animal, the significance of his observation was missed, though he underlined it with the remarkable sentence "it would be interesting to know whether an emulsion of thyroid gland would not have an analogous effect". We may presume that the effects of transplantation might have been interpreted as the replacement of a missing excretory organ, but the failure to follow up Schiff's further suggestion for six years shows how foreign the idea of internal secretion was to scientific thought of the day. Then in 1890 Vessale gave intravenous injections of thyroid extract to thyroidectomised dogs with beneficial results. The credit for the clinical application of this must be given to G. R. Murray, who had been House Physician at University College Hospital and met Horsley then. Murray wrote to Horsley, making the suggestion that myxoedema might be successfully treated by similar injections, but Horsley was not at first favourable to the idea. Indeed, he

(7)

said that the results so far obtained might have been caused by injection from any other tissue. Murray, at a meeting of the Northumberland and Durham Medical Society, showed a patient with myxoedema on whom he proposed to try this treatment. He received a douche of cold water, and later actual opposition. In no way deterred, he carried out his idea, with what success is now common knowledge. Horsley was converted, and a year later Hector Mackenzie and others simplified the treatment by giving thyroid by the mouth, thus establishing the discovery beyond cavil.

In 1894 Horsley was awarded a medal by the Royal Society "for his investigations relating to the physiology of the nervous system, and of the thyroid gland". These were of course two separate lines of enquiry, but my purpose today is to show under the title of "The Integration of the Endocrine System" how much more closely these two subjects are related than was imagined at that time.

It seems to me particularly appropriate to do so in this College, which has played so large a part in elucidating these problems, largely owing to the work and inspiration of Sir Edward Sharpey-Schäfer, whose recent passing away at a ripe old age, full of honours, leaves a notable gap in our ranks. For it was here that he with Oliver discovered the effects of adrenal and pituitary extracts; it was here that Bayliss and Starling discovered secretin, and it was here that Starling did the work that led him to enunciate the theory of hormones in his Croonian Lectures of 1905. Appropriately enough it was to you that Professor T. R. Elliott came from Cambridge, already distinguished for his researches on adrenalin. And to come down to recent days, it was here that Professor Harington proved the chemical structure of thyroxin. It is a record of which any institution may indeed be proud.

I would stress three recent lines of advance which are leading to a clearer conception of the integration of the endocrine system:

1. The diencephalon (particularly the hypothalamus) has been conclusively shown to be the nervous structure concerned with the expression of the emotions.

2. The pituitary, which is so closely associated

(9)   2

with the diencephalon, has become recognised as the leader of the endocrine orchestra.

3. It is now realised that all nervous impulses have a chemical mediator between the neuron and the tissue cell, and indeed between one neuron and another.

I shall proceed to expatiate on each of these three points in turn, and shall hope to show how they are leading to a new conception of the unity of functioning of the body.

1. From the experiments of Sherrington it has been known that if the higher parts of the brain be severed from the diencephalon in a dog, the animal responds to ordinary stimuli in an exaggerated way by an explosion of what he terms "sham rage". Cushing has reported similar explosions in a patient suffering from a cerebral tumour which similarly destroyed these connections.

The ravages of lethargic encephalitis on this part of the brain may not only damage the statics of the body but may profoundly affect the temperament and behaviour of the victim.

In these instances we are dealing with partial lesions which no doubt have an irritative effect on the remainder. But I will now refer to an extra-ordinary case under the care of Professor Naish[1] of Sheffield, in which a teratoma involving the whole of the hypothalamus completely blotted out the normal expression of the emotions; in Hughlings Jackson's nomenclature, a destroying rather than a discharging lesion.

A girl aged 10 came under observation with the following history. From birth she had been of an unusual temperament; the contrast being made more manifest to her parents after the birth of the second child who had normal reactions. As an infant she used to sleep considerably longer hours than the average for her age, and during her sleep she would never move. As she grew older it was noticed that she was very undemonstrative in the expression of emotions; she never showed joy or excitement. She never showed fear in the usual way, although she apparently felt fear, especially of loud noises, darkness, solitude, and certain persons. She would tell her parents that she was afraid, but her expression and voice were calm.

What was taken to be anger was shown by sudden refusal to comply with suggestions.

With this absence of expressiveness she yet appeared to have strong feelings, but she displayed none of the usual childish graces and her manners to chance callers were apparently rude. In this respect she appeared to be incorrigible and even unconscious of defect. She was very impenetrable to suggestion, and was what her parents called "strong-willed".

All her life she was liable to frequent sudden rises of temperature followed shortly by sudden falls. Her mental powers were good and she had an excellent memory. Her balance when walking or standing was never very good; when she tripped she seemed to have less than the usual powers of recovery and would fall flat on the floor.

Three years before her death it was noticed that she was drinking heavily and passing large quantities of pale urine both day and night. This was associated with a poor appetite for solid food and wasting; from this time she appeared not to grow at all. The polyuria continued up to about five weeks before her death and then ceased somewhat abruptly. There was no sugar in the urine. It was noticed that her emotional reactions were further diminished; she never shed a tear. Some three or four weeks before her death she found that she was unable to walk, and spontaneously surmised that she was going to die; she said in an indifferent tone, "Well, we can't help it".

She appeared to feel the cold intensely, and would do all she could to huddle in front of a big fire. This sensation steadily became worse and during the summer of 1933, which was exceptionally hot, she would wear an overcoat at meals. This feeling of cold ceased abruptly some two or three weeks before death. During this same summer it was noticed that she had begun to fall asleep in unusual places. Her powers of vision were lost apparently quite rapidly about five weeks before her death.

On admission she was remarkably drowsy. The pupils were equal and reacted normally. No cranial nerve paralysis was found; the reflexes were normal. There was marked pallor of the central area of each optic disc. She became comatose and died a few days later.

At the post-mortem a firm tumour with a smooth lobulated surface was found projecting from the base of the brain in the hypothalamic region behind the optic chiasma. The body showed no other abnormality except for enlargement of the mesenteric glands with evidence of tuberculous infection. The pituitary gland appeared to be normal.

Microscopically the tumour consisted of irregularly scattered epithelial elements in a connective tissue stroma. Bands of smooth muscle formed a prominent feature. The epithelial elements were frequently in the form of glandular spaces bounded by columnar cells. In one area there was an arrangement of epithelial cells closely resembling foetal glomeruli. In short it was a teratoma.

She therefore had temporary symptoms presumably due to pituitary compression, such as polyuria, disturbances of temperature and much drowsiness, but the most striking feature of the case was the blotting out of nearly all normal emotional expression.

There is then abundant evidence on the first

(14)

point. We pass to the second which really contains two separate propositions:

(a) The close association between the nervous diencephalon and the glandular pituitary.

The anatomists of the past, looking at the brain enclosed in bone, and joined by a narrow stalk to this small pituitary body also thus enclosed, like a brain in miniature, were struck with the idea of a little shrunken brain, which, as it were, responded to, or repeated, the actions of the big brain above. Modern research has shown that there is more in this idea than was supposed in the nineteenth century. Harvey Cushing, to whom more than any other one man our knowledge of the pituitary is due, gave a brilliant review in his Lister Memorial Lecture[2] of the relationship between this gland and the diencephalon lying immediately above it; he re-echoed the saying of Ridley in 1695 that "it seems in a manner almost impossible to treat of one independently of the other". The following quotations from his lecture may well serve to illustrate my point:

No other single structure of the body is so doubly protected, so centrally placed, so well hidden [as the pituitary]. Here in this well concealed spot, almost to be covered by a thumb-nail, lies the very mainspring of primitive existence—vegetative, emotional and reproductive—on which, with more or less success, man, chiefly, has come to superimpose a cortex of inhibitions. The symptoms arising from disturbance of this ancestral apparatus are beginning to stand out in their true significance. . . . The diencephalon is an ancient part of the brain which remains essentially unaltered in all creatures that have a brain at all. Moreover, it proves to have direct connections with the first of the organs of internal secretion to become recognisably differentiated, and on which the very perpetuation of the species depends. Such primitive instincts as hunger, thirst and sleep also seem to be mediated through this region. Cyclicism, which may be diurnal, lunar or seasonal, is a peculiarity of many physiological processes, such as oestrus, menstruation, hibernation and indeed ordinary sleep. That these processes are somehow under the control of the diencephalo-pituitary apparatus seems most probable. . . . Recent investigations serve closely to relate the diencephalon to metabolic processes, to the primary emotions and lastly to the sympathetic nervous system.

A clear cut instance of inhibition of the secretion of pituitrin through emotional disturbance is provided by Leslie Pugh's observation on cows that refuse to yield their milk, either because the calf has been taken away or because they object to an individual dairyman. If she hears the blaring of the calf the mother may yield her milk, but either cause of her refusal can be overcome by an injection of pituitrin. The disturbance of her diencephalon inhibits the chemical stimulus to the expulsion of milk, but the injection of that stimulant cuts under the nervous inhibition, and the milk perforce has to flow.

Diabetes insipidus has been referred by some observers to a hypothalamic lesion and by others to a pituitary one. It is generally admitted now that damage to either place or the stalk connecting them can have this effect. Since pitressin can reduce the secretion of water by a denervated kidney, it is clear that when a nerve lesion leads to polyuria it does so by interfering with the secretion of pitressin. Presumably nervous polyuria is a temporary functional condition of the same sort. Thus we may accept the view of a diencephalo-pituitary apparatus, in which the nervous apparatus can implement itself through the chemical secretions of the glandular portion. Moreover, as Herring has pointed out, this secretion may be diverted either into the hypothalamus or into the general circulation by a local vascular adjustment.

Having thus established the connection between the activities of the diencephalon and the pituitary, we may proceed to establish:

(b) That the pituitary is the leader of the endocrine orchestra. Cushing some years ago laid down the principle that polyglandular syndromes had their primary focus in some pituitary disturbance. The close association between the pituitary and the other endocrine glands is now generally admitted. Facts have accumulated so rapidly, that in order to gain any clear impression of the present position it is necessary to be concise and rather dogmatic. We recognise three types of cell in the anterior pituitary—the chromophobe which resists staining, the eosinophile and the basophile. The chromophobe is probably the parent cell of the other two. An adenoma composed of chromophobe cells diminishes pituitary function. Fröhlich's syndrome of obesity of the limb-girdle type and genital hypoplasia was originally recognised in a case of this sort. But extreme obesity may also result merely from division of the pituitary stalk either experimentally or by disease. Milder cases occur without the presence of an adenoma. They may be attributed to a delay in the differentiation of these chromophobe cells; puberty may be delayed but the outlook is not so serious. That the eosinophile cells are the source of a growth hormone can be definitely accepted. The experimental evidence as to the production of gigantism in rats, the clinical evidence derived from acromegaly and acromicry, from Simmonds' disease both in children and in adults, seem alike satisfactory, though Novak[3] maintains that this hormone has not yet been obtained free from all the others. The basophile cells became regarded as the source of the sex hormone after the researches of Evans and Simpson, and still more so after Cushing's description of the syndrome of pituitary basophilism.[4] We may accept the view that the growth and sex hormones are antagonistic, and that it is not until the latter gains the upper hand that puberty occurs, but as I hope to show later, there are strong reasons to doubt the basophile cells as the source of the sex hormone. The position with regard to gonadotropic hormones is decidedly involved. We must distinguish clearly between oestrogenic substances which can act directly in the absence of the ovaries and gonadotropic principles which act indirectly by exciting the production of oestrin in the ovary. It must always be remembered that the gonadotropic extracts in therapeutic use are obtained not from the pituitary but from the placenta or from pregnancy urine; their active principle is probably chorionic in origin. Although it is similar to, if not identical with, the type which can be obtained by chemical treatment of the pituitary, there is an important difference in their physiological action; the one obtained from the pituitary can produce both maturation of the ovarian follicles and their subsequent luteinisation in an animal deprived of its own pituitary, while the chorionic one cannot do either under such conditions (Collip[5]). The contrast between the small amount of oestrogenic substance produced by the pituitary and the enormous amount of oestrin found in the placenta, whence it overflows freely into the urine during pregnancy, is highly suggestive of a catalytic agent acting on a large mass of substrate, or at any rate of a stimulating synergic mechanism. In other words, while we must admit the prime importance of the anterior pituitary in initiating the events of the reproductive cycle, the process suggests that it does so by calling into activity hormones formed in the gonadal apparatus itself. This seems all the more probable in view of its capacity to evoke a response in male and female alike. More surprising is the fact that though the primary sex hormones are not identical, even though chemically closely related, descent of the testes in cryptorchids has been repeatedly observed after the injection of the extract from pregnancy urine.

It is still a matter of dispute whether the maturation and the luteinisation of an ovarian follicle are excited by two distinct hormones from the anterior pituitary or by only one, which produces these two effects according to the stage of the cycle. Most observers now, except Collip, seem to incline to the latter view, which would harmonise with the general conception I am advancing.

After the recognition of the growth and sex hormones, claims for other hormones secreted by the anterior pituitary multiplied rapidly. I will deal briefly with the principal ones.

The thyrotropic hormone. The loss of the secretion of the anterior pituitary through disease or experimental extirpation is followed by atrophy of the thyroid with reduction of the basal metabolic rate, and these changes can be prevented by injection of an anterior pituitary extract. Such an extract can produce hyperplasia of the thyroid with exophthalmos and an increased basal metabolic rate, but the two last named cannot be thus produced in animals from which the thyroid has been removed.[6] We have here an experimental method of producing Graves' disease, and as in the case of Graves' disease the condition can be controlled by the administration of iodine. Such observations throw light on the emotional causation of hyperthyroidism. It has long been known that the thyroid has an abundant supply of sympathetic nerves, but as these appear to be purely vasomotor, and indeed vasoconstrictor in action, it was difficult to see how their stimulation could lead to thyroid hypertrophy. It is therefore tempting to attribute such enlargement to excessive production of the thyrotropic hormone in the pituitary under diencephalic stimulation. Harington, however, thinks that although the greatly increased rate of secretion by the gland in hyperthyroidism is probably due to some extrinsic stimulus, and although the thyrotropic hormone has been shown to be such a potential cause, it is unlikely that anything so simple as the over-production of this hormone can account for Graves' disease.

Parathyrotropic hormone. It cannot be said that the case for the existence of a separate pituitary hormone affecting the parathyroids is established yet, but the striking similarity of the decalcification and bone pains of pituitary basophilism and of hyperparathyroidism is suggestive, despite the fact that in the former the blood calcium is not increased as in the latter.

Diabetogenic hormone. As is well known, and as

has now been amply confirmed, Houssay found that if a dog is previously deprived of its pituitary, subsequent removal of its pancreas does not cause glycosuria. But if an anterior pituitary extract is injected, the blood sugar is raised and sugar appears in the urine. Houssay has recently obtained this blood-sugar raising principle from the urine, and according to Wilder and Wilbur it acts by way of the adrenals on the liver. In this connection it is of great interest that Hertz[7] found symptoms of von Gierke's disease in a pituitary dwarf, suggesting that the non-utilisation of glycogen characteristic of that condition is due to a lack of Houssay's pituitary hormone. We are now realising the complexity of the endocrine-autonomic mechanism by which the blood-sugar level is maintained; a balance being struck between the agencies tending to depress it, *i.e.* the pancreas under the influence of the vagus, and those tending to raise it, *i.e.* both lobes of the pituitary, the thyroid and the adrenals acting with the sympathetic, while mid-brain and bulbar centres regulate the whole. Just as cerebral anaemia leads to a rise of blood pressure through peripheral vasoconstriction, and as increased hydrogen-ion concentration in the medulla leads to increased respiratory effort, so a fall of blood sugar brings into play the vagal mechanisms which raise it again. Conversely the intravenous injection of hypertonic glucose may so stimulate the other side of the balance that actual hypoglycaemia may follow.

It is an interesting fact that this Houssay hormone acts much more rapidly if injected into the cerebrospinal fluid according to Lucke, who regards this as evidence that it acts through the nervous centres and then presumably via the splanchnics on the adrenals. This is not unlike the view expressed by J. J. R. Macleod in the Herter lectures shortly before his death. Funk and others, noting the marked ketonuria which occurs both with Houssay's extract and in von Gierke's disease, claim to have isolated a separate *ketogenic principle*. They consider that it is not identical with the one that raises blood sugar because it increases the lipoid content of the blood, which the latter does not do. And so the multiplication of hormones goes on, and there is now added a

Lactogenic hormone. It has long been recognised that the postpituitary can influence the expulsion of milk from the mammary ducts, but it is now claimed that an anterior pituitary hormone, pro-lactin, stimulates the actual secretion, while oestrin is responsible for the unfolding of the mammary duct system.[8]

Adrenotropic hormone. Here we are on rather securer ground. The close resemblance between pituitary and adrenal virilism, the fact that progeria was first referred to adrenal atrophy and now to atrophy of the pituitary, the association of anencephaly with incomplete development of the adrenals all point to some fairly close inter-action. Experimentally, injection of anterior pituitary extracts can produce marked adrenal hypertrophy. Among others, Vines and Broster, Lescher and Robb-Smith[9] have emphasised the great difficulty of determining whether in a case of virilism the primary lesion is in the pituitary or the adrenal. Indeed, in proved cases of a pituitary basophile adenoma such as Parkes Weber's, the adrenals showed hypertrophy.

The rôle of the basophile cells. We are now in a

position to come to closer grips with the questions —what is the function of the basophile cells and can we draw any conclusions therefrom which will throw light on the way in which the pituitary does its work? We were a little too ready to conclude that the syndrome of pituitary baso-philism confirmed the idea that the sex hormone originated in the basophile cells. Woollard[10] was the first, as far as I am aware, to point out that if this were so, it is unreasonable to suppose that in women virilism and decay of sexual function should follow excess of it. Injection of pituitary gonadotropic hormone produces nothing like pituitary basophilism, but may produce gonadal atrophy. He therefore does not believe that the basophile cells are the source of the sex hormone; rather, he envisages them as the inhibitors of the acidophilic activities. He thinks the evidence warrants the statement that the pituitary plays no part in sexual differentiation, but exerts its effects on either the testis or the ovary, bringing each to its structural differentiation and to its full endocrine activity. Lescher and Robb-Smith come to a similar conclusion, that the basophile

(27)

cells are the source of some depressive inhibitory substance. Levy Simpson[11] also suggests that the basophile secretion is inhibitory on the homosexual glands, allowing the development of a latent heterosexual rudiment. It is true that Wright has reported an excess of the pituitary sex hormone in the urine of female patients with basophilism, though Levy Simpson thinks it is the male sex hormone that is present. In any case clinical evidence of increased sexual activity in such patients is, to say the least, more than dubious.

Crooke[12] has described a characteristic hyaline change in the basophile cells in Cushing's syndrome, whether that syndrome be associated with basophilic adenoma or a neoplasm of the thymus or hyperplasia or a neoplasm of the adrenal cortex. He did not regard this as a degenerative change, but as an expression of altered physiological activity. In Addison's disease he, in conjunction with Dorothy Russell,[13] found an extreme reduction in the pituitary basophile cells. They think this may be the cause of the low blood pressure and possibly of the hypoglycaemia in this disease; it is certainly in sharp contrast with the high pressure and hyperglycaemia found with basophilic adenomas. These two authors together with Horace Evans [14] have described two cases of such adenomas in which most of the characteristic symptoms of the syndrome were lacking, cardio-vascular hypertrophy being the salient feature. Nevertheless they are not prepared to go as far as Cushing in regarding essential hypertension as due to increase in the number of basophile cells. Broster and Vines regard an excess of fuchsin staining material as the essential change in the adrenal cortical cells which produces virilism. This change may be absent in pituitary baso-philism. The way in which a growth in the thymus gland, usually regarded as antagonistic to sexual development, may stimulate the basophilic syn-drome adds to all these doubts concerning the sexual functions of the basophile cells.

In earlier days the number of "centres" located by the physiologist in the medulla around the fourth ventricle multiplied until they produced a revolt against the whole conception. That centres should exist ready-made for a contingency which might never arise throughout life was a *reductio ad absurdum*. In the same way the functions controlled by the anterior pituitary have multiplied until the existence of a separate hormone for each function has become almost incredible. As P. E. Smith[15] puts it: "That this small gland, which in man averages less than half a gram in weight, secretes this number of hormones as separate entities throughout the entire secretory process taxes the imagination. The differentiation into two highly specialised secretory types suggests perhaps the formation of a corresponding number of basic secretory products which may be altered to give these specific responses. There can be no certainty until physiologically pure extracts are secured as to how much these impurities may modify the response." One might add to this the fact that somewhat violent chemical measures have been adopted to isolate these pituitary hormones even in only an approximately pure state. It seems more probable that such measures have produced alterations in the basic products as P. E. Smith suggests. In the less complicated case of the thyroid Harington[16] believes that the molecule of the complete active secretion contains both thyroxin and diiodotyrosine, and that some linkage between them is ruptured during the hydrolysis necessary for the isolation of thyroxin. Surely something of the same sort is probable in the case of the pituitary. Thus its thyrotropic hormone is obtained by acid extraction, which may easily produce changes in chemical structure.

In view of these facts, this newer conception of the anterior pituitary producing an accelerating hormone in the eosinophile cells and an inhibitory one in the basophile cells seems a rational one—the functions and the staining reactions of these cells being alike diametrically opposed. One may regard the anterior pituitary as largely controlled by the diencephalon and putting down the loud or soft pedal, as it were, on the other glands.

Fresh light on the whole subject has been thrown by Dodds[17], who classifies hormones under two headings. The first are complex protein bodies formed by the anterior pituitary, which act on the other endocrine glands causing them to form the secondary type of hormones which are bodies of comparatively small molecular weight, most of which have been isolated in a crystalline form and some of which have actually been prepared synthetically. It will be noted that in this respect the posterior pituitary belongs to the second group.

In conjunction with Cook he has carried out a brilliant series of researches into these secondary hormones and has shown that simpler compounds than those prepared by the body can have the same biological effect to a less or even greater extent. This basal group with the simplest chemical structure that can produce the biological effect he calls the "skeleton key" which picks the physiological lock. Even more striking was his demonstration that the same basal group could produce more than one biological effect. To such groups he gave the name of "pass keys". Perhaps the most impressive instance of this is the condensation of benzene rings into a phenanthrene ring which by simple alteration in the degree of hydrogenation can give rise to oestrin, to Vitamin D or calciferol, and to the carcinogenetic substance present in coal tar. It is accordingly by no means fanciful to regard the anterior pituitary as receiving the impulses from the diencephalon, and producing an activating and an inhibitory hormone of a protein character according to demand, which can speed up or inhibit the secretion of the simpler grade of hormone in the other endocrine glands; hormones which are of allied chemical structure and which in some instances may even be interchangeable in their action. At any rate it is a unifying hypothesis which deserves further and careful consideration.

Antihormones. The question has not been simplified by the claims made for the existence of antihormones. Collip showed some time ago that parathormone gradually lost its effect on repeated injections. One might imagine that this failure could be adequately accounted for by its destructive action on the calcium content of bone and muscle, but he now[18] thinks that there is an antihormone both to the pituitary growth and thyrotropic hormones, and advances the hypothesis that the production of antihormones may be responsible for hypoglandular states. He regards a hormone-antihormone linkage as the normal condition, which can readily be disturbed.

The purposive character of such antihormones is hard to see; certainly thyroid administration is effective when continued over many years. The claim for the existence of a catechin in the blood which is antagonistic to thyroxin, if substantiated, suggests a simpler explanation, namely that various chemical substances can destroy hormones, just as we know the acetylcholine and adrenaline set free on nerve stimulation are rapidly destroyed in the blood or tissue cells.

And this leads me directly to my third point. It has long been common knowledge that emotional states may modify secretion; the tears of sorrow and the dry mouth of fear are proverbial. In such instances it is obvious that a nervous impulse has produced or prevented a chemical process. But it is only quite recently that we have realised that *all nervous impulses have a chemical mediator between the neuron and the tissue cell, and indeed between one neuron and another.* In Hopkins' phrase, chemical substances are produced which translate for the tissues the messages received by nerves. We have indeed been curiously blind to the fact that the chemical changes produced in a gland by nervous stimulation is only a special case of a general law. I say curiously blind, because this century was only about one year old when Langley found a clue which was not really followed up for years. We knew that adrenaline is manufactured by the cells of the adrenal medulla, which are actually formed out of sympathetic ganglion cells. Langley enunciated the law that the effect of adrenaline on any part is the same as if the sympathetic nerves to that part were stimulated; an extraordinarily interesting example of a chemical substance imitating a nervous response. The adrenal medulla was seen to represent the postganglionic element in the sympathetic. In 1907 W. E. Dixon made some tentative experiments on the liberation of a chemical substance in the heart after vagus stimulation; unfortunately this encountered so much scepticism that he dropped the subject. But later the work of Loewi and of Dale has proved that acetylcholine is liberated at the terminals whenever sympathetic or parasympathetic preganglionic fibres are stimulated, and adrenaline at the sympathetic postganglionic terminals. So Dale[19] speaks of

(35)

cholinergic and adrenergic fibres, and incidentally shows how this conception explains Langley and Anderson's cross-suturing experiments. You can cross-suture cholinergic with cholinergic or adrenergic with adrenergic, but you cannot successfully cross-suture cholinergic with adrenergic fibres. Cannon thinks that the substance liberated at the sympathetic postganglionic terminal is not identical with adrenaline; he thinks he can extract a slightly different one after an excitant action from that appearing after an inhibitory one. But is it not possible that the adrenaline is modified by an ergotoxin-like action in the former case? For Loewi has shown that physostigmine imitates or increases the effect of parasympathetic stimulation because it prevents the blood or the tissue cell from destroying the acetylcholine produced. Just as physostigmine facilitates, so does atropine interfere with the normal chemical results of parasympathetic stimulation. It is important to note that just as much acetylcholine is produced whether atropine is given or not—the atropine merely blocks access to the tissue cell.

This leads me to an aspect of endocrinology

which is urgently demanding attention. Some thirty years ago Langley and Elliott independently postulated the existence of a receptive substance between the nerve ending and the tissue as necessary to explain the facts then known. If such a postulate was required then, how much more is it needed today? Just as the appropriate chemical material may get into this receptive substance, so may a toxin. G. N. Myers has shown that a therapeutic drug may seize on the receptive substance and thus bar the way to the ingress of the toxin. It seems to me that the pharmacology of the future will have to concern itself with the natural history of these receptive substances, and find out in what way they can be helped by drugs both positively, by facilitating their reactions, and negatively, by blocking the way against the entrance of toxins. Nor is this topic remote from my subject, for Zondek maintains that the adsorption of a hormone such as thyroxin is decreased in the presence of narcotics, such as the barbiturates, which are able to adhere to the cell surface and thus to displace the hormone from it. But it is also germane to my subject in a wider sense. Sir Henry Dale in his recent Harveian Oration before the Royal College of Physicians [20] reminded us that we are still entirely without any conception why a particular cell should be sensitive to a particular chemical substance or why the same substance should augment the activity of one type of cell and inhibit that of another. He indicates indeed precisely the problem to which many minds are beginning to devote themselves, the nature of these receptive substances. The nature of the stimulus has been intensively studied, but it is now clear that this is only half, and perhaps the simpler half of the question. The importance of the responsive capacity of the receptor tissues was clearly indicated by Harrison in his Harvey Lectures for 1934. He showed that when transplantation is effected between embryos of species of different sizes, the transplant responds according to its inherited growth capacity rather than to its new endocrine environment. As Keith pointed out some years ago, the partial gigantisms in certain cases of hyperpituitarism can only be explained on the theory that the locally hypertrophied tissues had devolved a special sensitiveness to the growth hormone. H. M. Evans[21] has recently shown that the response of the dachshund and of the sheep dog to injections of the pituitary growth hormone is entirely different. Indeed, if such things were not so, it would be difficult to account for the structural plasticity of the dog in the hands of the breeder.

Again, after the menopause oestrin may be present in large amounts yet reproductive cycles cease, as if the reproductive organs had lost their capacity to respond rather than that the hormonic stimulus had failed.[22] According to Zondek, the fact that hormones in such minute quantities can produce marked generalised effects indicates that they act as catalysts; their activity seems apparently to depend upon the integrity of cellular structure; they are *physical* catalysts. He maintains that the hormones circulate in the blood in an inactive form; not until they reach the organ of their destination, where they are adsorbed, do they become activated. But at present we have no inkling as to the mechanisms by which any such cellular response is produced or rendered specific. Hopkins,[23] commenting on the comparative failure of the attempts to correlate chemical structure with pharmacological action, pointed out that so far the investigation had been one-sided and should involve consideration of the structure of the cell. The same comment is applicable to the present position of endocrinology.

For a time after Starling developed his conception of the chemical control of the body by hormones, the pendulum swung so far in that direction that it seemed as if the nervous system would be deprived of its pride of place, although Starling himself had pointed out that its special function was to provide for special rapidity of response when required. There are a good many examples of a double mechanism in physiology, and it might be expected to occur in the endocrine system. Cannon's theory of the emergency action of adrenalin in coming to the assistance of the defensive apparatus of the sympathetic is a good example, which, though seriously criticised by Stewart and Rogoff, seems to have re-established itself in favour. Indeed, Dale's work makes it all the more intelligible and probable. Then the

(40)

nervous control over the pancreatic secretions, both external and internal, became recognised in addition to chemical methods of stimulation such as secretin. If the recent claims [24] are substantiated, that the oral administration of a duodenal extract can keep the blood sugar of a diabetic normal after he has first been treated by insulin, not only will this double mechanism have been proved for the internal secretion of the pancreas but a therapeutic advance of importance will have been made. And so the pendulum is swinging back again. But lest it should be thought that the propositions with which I started stressed the nervous control too much, I will try and restore the balance by referring to recent work on the organiser in the embryo.

We have realised for years that lowly organisms react to such stimuli as light and chemical agents at an evolutionary level before a central nervous system has appeared. But recent embryological work has shown the profound influence exerted by chemical agents on the very genesis of the nervous system. Some twelve years ago Spéman showed that if he transplanted a group of cells from the dorsal lip of the blastopore, *i.e.* the part where a central nervous system would first appear in the development, to some other part of an embryo, it would lead to the initiation of a central nervous system there, however different the situation was from the normal one. He could produce two central nervous systems at right angles to each other. He called these cells the organiser. Recently the Needhams and Waddington[25] at Cambridge have shown that they can reproduce all the effects of the organiser by extracting a chemical substance from these cells which resists both freezing and boiling. It is therefore a very definite chemical entity but not a ferment. Thus from the very start chemical and nervous mechanisms are interdependent. They have now gone on to some most exciting observations. They have been able to imitate this chemical organiser synthetically and it appears to be closely allied to, if not identical with, oestrin, which we know to be a sterol. Thus the ovarian hormone is apparently carried on to the next generation and is primarily responsible for organising the central nervous system. These observers have also been

(42)

able in a similar way to lead to the formation of various mesodermal structures in parts of the body to which they are foreign.

It seems to me probable that the formation of teratomata is to be explained by the escape of such chemical organisers from their proper site. Dr Needham has called my attention to some observations by Witschi [26] on the results of delaying the fertilisation of amphibian ova. If the sperm cell is not allowed to unite with the egg cell almost at once, there is a disturbance of the normal sex-ratio in the offspring. If there is a further delay the organiser is liberated at the wrong time and place and teratomata result. Finally, if there is a still greater delay exceedingly abnormal monsters result which actually produce metastases when implanted into adult amphibia. Holtfreter in Munich has already applied these results to the explanation of teratomata in human beings.

It would be a valuable piece of gynaecological research to see if the occurrence of maternal salpingitis or endometritis, which might well delay the fertilisation of the egg cell, could be correlated with the incidence of teratomata. But it would be difficult because a teratoma may produce no symptoms for years. However, Aschheim[27] states that the gonadotropic hormone of pregnancy is to be found in the urine of patients suffering from a teratoma, even in the case of a man! This may provide a diagnostic test of real value, and seems to make still more probable the association of teratomata with oestrin gone astray, as it were. Incidentally I may suggest that the discovery of the importance of oestrin for the development of the embryo may explain why the chorionic villi of the placenta should manufacture it in such large amounts. For hitherto I do not know that a reason has been given for this striking fact.

That oestrin, calciferol and the carcinogenetic substance in coal tar should all be closely related sterols is remarkably interesting. It is extraordinary to find that the necessary stimuli to the growth of the next generation, to the ordinary growth of bone and to the disorderly growth of malignant disease are due to closely similar chemical substances. That they should to some extent be interchangeable is even more extraordinary. The fact that teratomata stand half-way between abnormal twinning and malignancy is full of interest. It is true that some critics declare that to say that all these conditions are associated with alterations of sterol metabolism is no more than saying that another group of conditions are associated with altered protein metabolism, so manifold are the sterols. Loeb [28] is of opinion that though the hydrocarbons of tar and the oestrogenic hormones may be more efficient than other factors in producing cancer, in principle they do not act differently from numerous other conditions which may cause it. They seem able to induce the change at any point where they come into prolonged contact with tissues which still possess the potentiality of growth and proliferation. But I think such criticisms rather unnecessarily belittle a remarkable series of mutually consistent observations. The widespread importance of sterols in what one may call the metabolism of the moment has received additional evidence from some recent researches of Carter and Mapson,[29] who find that for the proper functioning of both voluntary and cardiac muscle in the frog, a definite proportion between the concentrations of acetylcholine and sterols in the tissue is necessary. They find moreover that many of the sterols can replace each other in this as in their other actions. Further, they showed that if thyroxin is added to the Ringer's solution in which the muscle is bathed, a tetanic contraction instead of the normal single twitch results on electrical stimulation if this acetylcholine-sterol balance is disturbed. Further unpublished work by them has shown that a similar balance between thyroid and antithyroid principles is necessary. Here are some hints as to the lines along which research may reveal something of the factors controlling the receptive mechanisms.

Before drawing the threads of my argument together, it may be well to say something on sex reversal in general, to which scattered allusions have been made in passing. Undoubtedly the initial bias in sex differentiation is determined by the chromosomes. But although this is the sole and efficient cause in, for instance, insects, its effect is much slighter in birds and mammals, and has to be reinforced by the endocrine activity proper to each sex. Indeed, as Woollard [30] has pointed out, before this time is reached the influence of the chromosomes is so weak that the embryo passes through an indifferent or bisexual phase. This is followed by a brief interval when a masculinising tendency apparently occurs in both sexes; in the female it declares itself as a medullary mass in the rete of the ovary which is really a testicular rudiment, and which may later in life become the site of a virilising new growth. The gonadal territory in the embryo consists in the first instance of a ridge on the medial side of the mesonephric mass. It seems certain that sex reversal is caused by an abnormal growth of mesonephric derivatives which are normally present, though only in a rudimentary form in the female. It follows that the testis is monosexual while the ovary is bisexual, with a male medulla and a female cortex, as it has been expressed. Therefore physical sex reversal can only occur in woman, and may be due to

1. Overaction of a basophilic adenoma which inhibits normal ovarian activity, allowing the rudimentary masculine elements to reassert themselves.

2. Overaction of the adrenal cortex, which is mesonephric and contains similar cells to those of the testis.

3. Overaction of mesonephric cells in the rete ovarii, which, as in some of the arrhenoblastomas first described by Pick,[31] may actually develop convoluted tubules resembling the seminiferous tubules of the testis.

Closely similar syndromes of virilism may originate in any one of these three positions and are all due to absolute or relative overaction of masculinising mesonephric structures. On the other hand, the testis being monosexual, sex reversal in man can only be psychogenic.

To state briefly the view of the integration of the endocrine system which I am attempting to visualise—there is doubtless an autonomous activity of these glands according to the steady biochemical demands of the body, but their activity can be profoundly modified and extensively controlled by centres in the diencephalon which are largely concerned with emotional expression. These centres may operate directly through the sympathetic nervous system (indeed the hypothalamus has been regarded by Beattie and others[32] as the head ganglion of the sympathetic) or indirectly through the chemical activities of the anterior pituitary. The anterior pituitary forms two basic secretions probably of a protein character, one being stimulating, the other inhibitory in effect. They correspond in fact to Sharpey-Schäfer's original distinction between a hormone and a chalone. It is suggested that the former is produced by the eosinophile, the latter by the basophile cells. These basic secretions are capable of chemical modification according to the needs of the body, and are then ready to stimulate or restrain the secretion of simpler hormones by the other endocrine glands including the post-pituitary. It may be, as Zondek[33] maintains, that the hormones circulate in an inactive form, only becoming activated when they reach their destination. This indeed might explain some of the observations on the alleged hormone-antihormone linkage. Certain it is that their destination is decided by some peculiar receptive capacity in the structure on which they act, catalytically or otherwise. What determines that receptive capacity we do not know as yet. But we can say that the whole process appears to be a special case of the general law that nervous stimuli, whether passing from the diencephalon to the pituitary, or down neurons to pre- and post-ganglionic endings, act through the intermediary of chemical substances locally produced. And we may find some further support for this view in the fact that, in one instance, the same substance, adrenaline, is the final product of either hormonic or nervous activity.

Historically it is interesting that in 1775 Bordeu wrote: "Every organ serves as a workshop for the preparation of a specific substance which enters into the blood; such substances are useful to the body, and are needed in order to maintain its integrity." Here indeed was the germ of the idea of internal secretion, which was however to lie dormant for more than a century. In its renaissance Victor Horsley played an important part, though at the outset he showed a caution not always characteristic of him. It is not merely for that reason that we are here assembled to do honour to his memory. It is of the man himself of whom we are thinking—attractive, vivid, eager, enthusiastic, a very Rupert of debate, and, may I say, an intellectual hormone in his effect upon others. Osler tells us that in October 1873 he listened to an introductory lecture at one of the largest of the London medical schools, the burden of which was that the art of surgery had all but reached its limits! In the falsification of that gloomy prognosis, Horsley with his pathological training, his new ideas, his fresh technique, must be allotted an honourable share. For all these reasons we honour his name and cherish his memory, and I in turn must offer my sincere thanks that it should have been entrusted to me to voice, however inadequately, your feelings on this occasion.

REFERENCES

1. H. E. Harding and A. E. Naish. *Lancet*, 1935, i, p. 77.
2. H. Cushing. *Lancet*, 1930, ii, pp. 119 and 175.
3. E. Novak. *J.A.M.A.* CIV, p. 998.
4. H. Cushing. *Arch. Int. Med.* LI, pp. 487–557.
5. J. B. Collip. *J.A.M.A.* CIV, p. 556.
6. J. B. Collip. *J.A.M.A.* CIV, p. 916. E. F. Scowen and A. W. Spence, *B.M.J.* 1934, ii, p. 805.
7. Quoted by Collip. *J.A.M.A.* CIV, p. 827.
8. P. E. Smith. *J.A.M.A.* CIV, p. 548.
9. F. G. Lescher and A. H. T. Robb-Smith. *Quart. Journ. Med.* Jan. 1935, p. 23.
10. H. H. Woollard. *Proc. Roy. Soc. Med.* XXVII, 1934, p. 271.
11. Levy Simpson. *Proc. Roy. Soc. Med.* (Clin. Sect.), 1933, p. 383.
12. A. C. Crooke. *Journ. Path. and Bact.* XLI, 1935, p. 339.
13. Dorothy Russell and A. C. Crooke. *Journ. Path. and Bact.* XL, 1935, p. 255.
14. D. Russell, H. Evans and A. C. Crooke. *Lancet*, 1934, ii, p. 240.
15. P. E. Smith. *Loc. cit.*
16. C. R. Harington. *Lancet*, 1925, i, pp. 1199 and 1261.
17. E. C. Dodds. *Lancet*, 1934, i, pp. 931, 987, 1048.

18. J. B. Collip. *J.A.M.A.* CIV, p. 965.
19. H. H. Dale. *Dixon Memorial Lecture*, 1934; *Linacre Lecture*, 1934.
20. H. H. Dale. *B.M.J.* Oct. 26, 1935.
21. Quoted by P. E. Smith. *Loc. cit.*
22. H. M. Evans. *J.A.M.A.* CIV, p. 464.
23. F. Gowland Hopkins. *Brit. Assoc. Presidential Address*, 1933.
24. G. G. Duncan *et al.* *Amer. Journ. Med. Sci.* CLXXXIX, p. 403.
25. J. Needham, C. H. Waddington and D. M. Needham. *Proc. Roy. Soc.* B, CXIV, 1934, p. 393.
26. E. Witschi. *Proc. Soc. Exp. Biol. and Med.* XXVII, 1930, p. 475 and XXXI, 1934, p. 419.
27. S. Aschheim. *J.A.M.A.* CIV, p. 1324.
28. L. Loeb. *J.A.M.A.* CIV, p. 1597.
29. Carter and Mapson. *Nature*, CXXXVI, 1935, p. 143.
30. H. H. Woollard. *Loc. cit.*
31. Pick. *Berl. Klin. Woch.* XIX, 1905, p. 502.
32. Beattie, Brow and Long. *Proc. Roy. Soc.* B, CVI, pp. 253-275.
33. H. Zondek. *The Diseases of the Endocrine Glands*, 3rd edit. London: Edward Arnold & Co. 1935, p. 8.